LOW ACID DIET COOKBOOK

Learn How to Cook Simple and Easy to make Low-Acid Delicious Meals without Triggering Acid Reflux, GERD, or LPR.

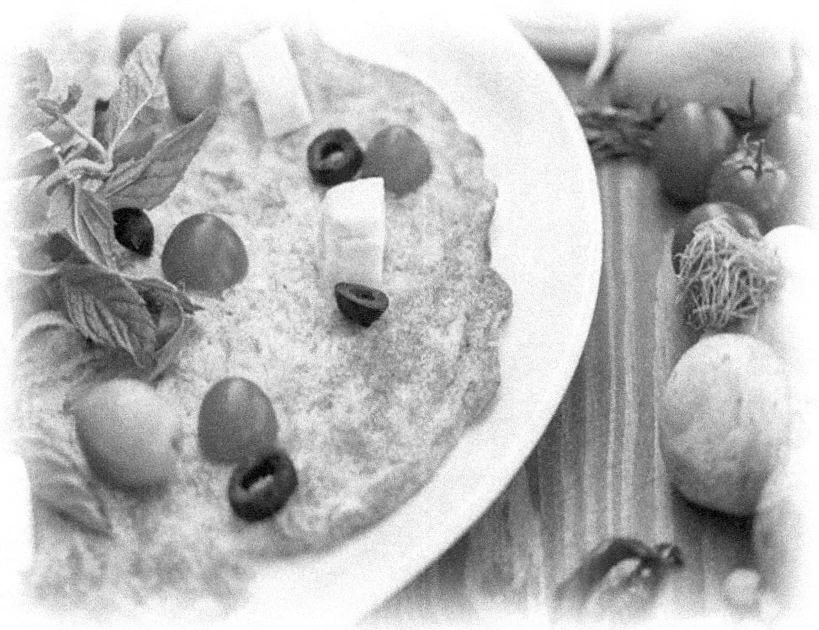

CHRISTIANA WHITE

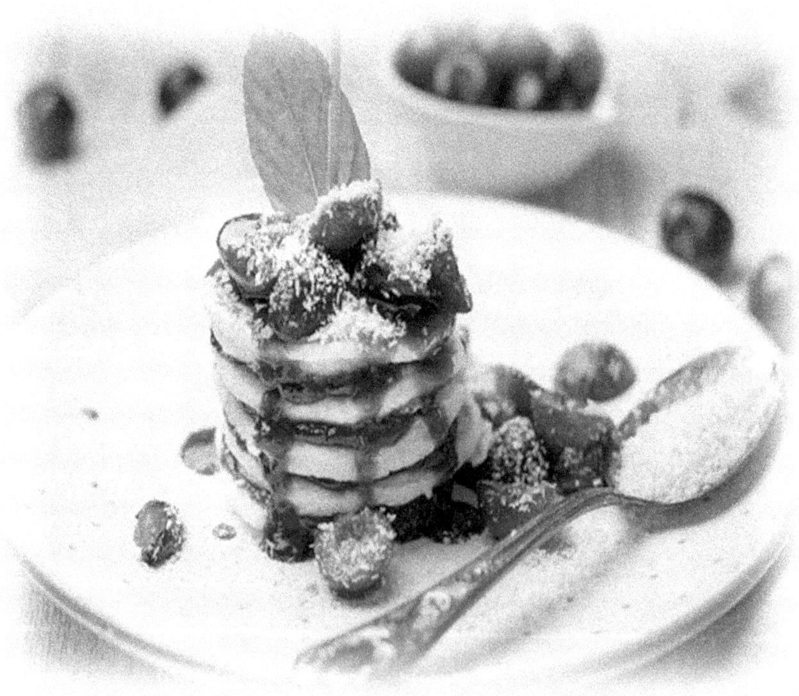

TABLE OF CONTENTS.

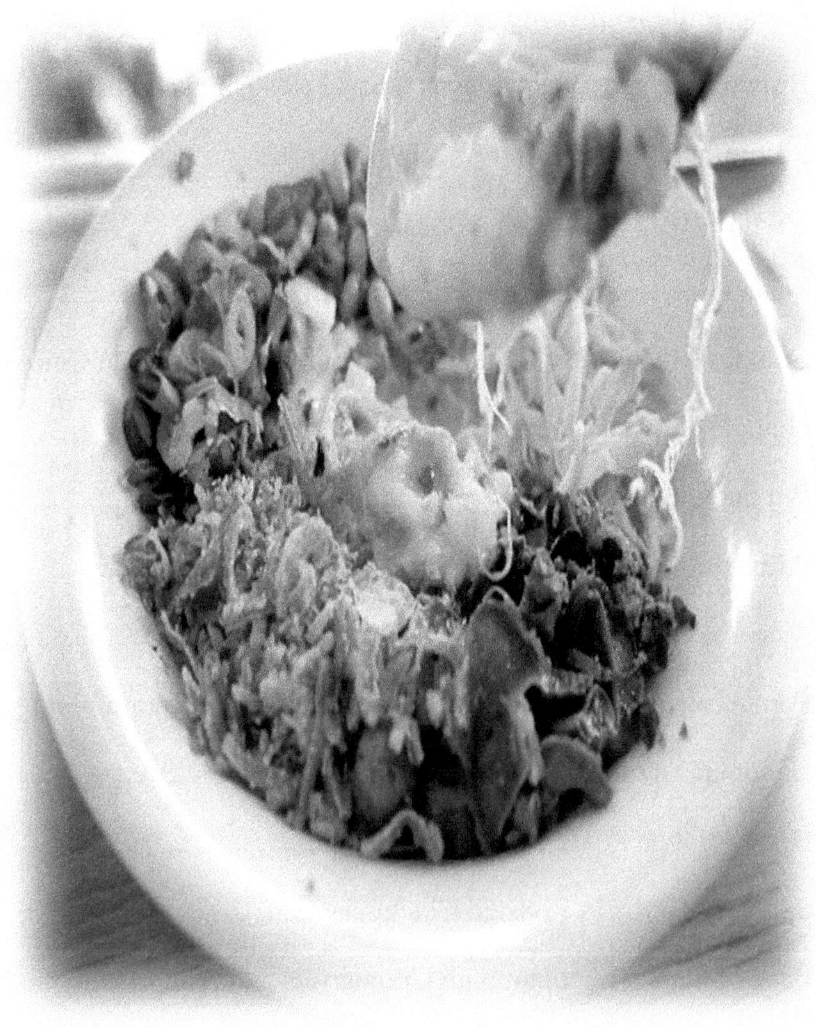

INTRODUCTION

Welcome to the Low Acid Diet Cookbook, a world of flavor without compromising, where taste and health come together beautifully. You're in the right place if you've ever craved for a culinary adventure that not only satisfies your taste senses but also promotes your wellbeing.

Throughout the process of creating this cookbook, we have seen countless people adopt a new eating style that celebrates scrumptious and healthful living while pushing the limits of dietary constraints. People from many walks of life have found resonance in this journey, and we can't wait to reveal the secret to you.

This is a testimonial to the transformational impact of the low-acid diet, not merely a compilation of recipes. We've witnessed how it's empowered people with GERD and acid reflux as well as those just trying to live a better lifestyle. The anecdotes we've heard are uplifting: tales of relishing meals free from the aches and pains caused by acidity, of consuming food that tantalizes the taste buds in addition to providing nourishment to the body.

Just picture yourself enjoying every bite of your favorite foods without worrying about causing acidity. Imagine a society in which eating healthily is a celebration of flavorful foods and nutritious components rather than a compromise. This is what the Low Acid Diet Cookbook is all about.

You'll find more than recipes when you turn the pages of these pages. You'll discover how to follow the guidelines of a low acid diet while constructing a low acid pantry, preparing breakfasts that make your day, savoring lunches and dinners, delighting in sweet treats, and drinking drinks that revitalize and refresh.

Thus, this cookbook is your reliable friend whether you're starting out on a healthy diet or looking to expand your repertoire of low-acid meals. Join the group of people who have embraced the Low Acid Diet Cookbook and discovered the delight of consuming scrumptious and healthful food.

The Advantages of Adopting a Lifestyle with Low Acidity

Eating foods that are low in acid, or alkaline, and avoiding meals that are high in acid, or acidic, is known as a low acid lifestyle. A low-acid lifestyle aims to bring the body's pH level, which indicates how acidic or alkaline it is, into equilibrium.

A pH of seven is considered neutral; a pH of less than seven is acidic, and a pH of more than seven is alkaline.

• It might aid in preventing or lessening acid reflux, a disorder that results in heartburn, irritation, and other symptoms when stomach acid escapes into the esophagus.

Foods and beverages high in acid, such as pizza, fried food, tomato sauce, citrus fruits, chocolate, coffee, and soda, can cause acid reflux.

You can prevent or lessen these triggers and lessen the frequency and intensity of acid reflux episodes by eating low-acid foods like whole grains, root vegetables, green vegetables, bananas, melons, cauliflower, fennel, nuts, celery, cucumber, lettuce, watermelon, broth-based soups, and herbal tea.

• As low-acid foods are easier for the body to digest and absorb, it might help with digestion and nutritional absorption. Foods high in acidity can disrupt the digestive enzymes, leading to indigestion, gas, bloating, constipation, diarrhea, and malnourishment.

Low-acid foods supply the body with vital vitamins, minerals, and antioxidants while also assisting the digestive system in operating more properly.

• Because low-acid meals are alkalizing and anti-inflammatory, they may strengthen your immune system and reduce inflammation.

Foods high in acid can cause the body to become acidic, which can impair immunity and exacerbate inflammation.

Numerous chronic illnesses, including diabetes, cancer, rheumatoid arthritis, asthma, and osteoporosis, are associated with inflammation. Foods low in acidity can support the body's natural pH balance, strengthening the immune system and lowering inflammation.

• Because low-acid meals are low in calories, fat, and sugar and high in fiber, water, and minerals, they may help with weight loss and prevent obesity. Foods with high acid content are frequently refined, processed, and heavy in calories, fat, and sugar, all of which can lead to weight gain and obesity.

Eat more foods low in acidity to help you feel fuller for longer and avoid overindulging.

Alkaline meals need more energy to process than acidic ones, so they can also help you burn more fat and calories.

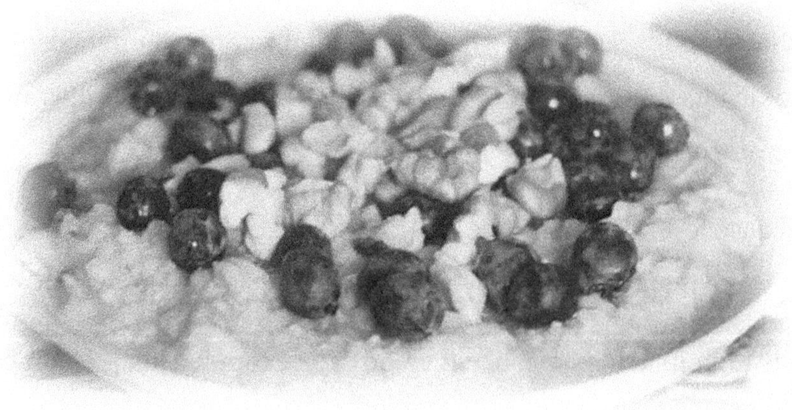

CHAPTER 1

Understanding the Low-Acid Diet

Introducing the Fundamentals

The goal of a low acid diet is to consume fewer foods and drinks that are high in acidity or that may aggravate acid reflux. Heartburn and other symptoms might result from acid reflux, a condition in which stomach acid refluxes back into the esophagus. By reducing the amount of acid in the stomach and esophagus, a low-acid diet can help avoid or treat these symptoms.

The following are a few meals and drinks that are thought to be acidic or that may cause acid reflux:

• Citrus fruits and liquids, including limes, oranges, lemons, and grapefruits

• Tomatoes and goods made with tomatoes, like ketchup, soups, and sauces

• Spicy dishes like curry, chile, garlic, and onions

• Fried and fatty meals including oils, cheese, bacon, and butter

• Peppermint, chocolate, and mint

• Tea, coffee, and beverages with caffeine

• Vinegar, carbonated beverages, and alcohol

You don't have to fully eliminate certain foods and drinks in order to follow a low acid diet; instead, you can restrict or moderate your intake of them.

Alternatives that are less acidic or less prone to result in acid reflux include:

• Fruits and juices that are not citrus, like pears, apples, bananas, and melons

• Vegetables, including spinach, celery, carrots, and broccoli

• Lean foods including fish, turkey, and chicken

• Whole grains, including quinoa, brown rice, and oats

• Dairy goods low in fat, like cheese, yogurt, and milk

• Herbal teas, including fennel, ginger, and chamomile

• Almond milk, water, and coconut water

There is no one-size-fits-all low-acid diet because everyone experiences acid reflux differently and has varying tolerances and triggers. As a result, it's critical to monitor your food and beverage intake and how it influences your symptoms.

You can keep track of your meals, snacks, and drinks using a food journal or an app. You can also record any symptoms of acid reflux, like heartburn, regurgitation, coughing, or sore throats. You can use this to determine your own triggers and modify your diet accordingly.

The Health Advantages of a Low-Acid Diet

A low-acid diet has several health advantages, particularly for those with acid reflux disease (GERD), laryngeal reflux disease (LPR), or Barrett's esophagus, among other disorders that are related to acid reflux.

• Diminishing the occurrence and intensity of acid reflux symptoms, like heartburn, chest discomfort, and sore throat

• Enhancing the well-being and quality of life of individuals who have acid reflux by allowing them to enjoy meals and activities without worrying about the discomfort and difficulties of the condition

• Avoiding or postponing the emergence of chronic acid reflux problems, such as cancer, esophagitis, ulcers, strictures, and bleeding.

• Encouraging the digestive system's general health and function since a low-acid diet can support a pH level that is balanced, a microbiome that is in good condition, and a robust mucosal barrier in the esophagus and stomach.

• Improving the nutritional status and intake of individuals with acid reflux, since a low-acid diet can promote the consumption of more fiber-rich whole grains, fruits, vegetables, and lean proteins.

In addition to improving overall health and wellness, a low-acid diet can help those without acid reflux avoid developing the condition altogether by delaying the onset of acid reflux and other digestive issues.

Because a low-acid diet can lessen oxidative stress, inflammation, and acidity in the body, it can benefit the immune system, cardiovascular system, neurological system, skin, and bones.

A low-acid diet is a balanced, diversified diet that may accommodate a range of tastes, interests, and lifestyles rather than being restricted or boring. A low-acid diet can provide a variety of meals and drinks that are low in acid or neutralize acid, making it tasty, fulfilling, and pleasurable.

• Whole wheat bread, tortillas, or pita bread stuffed with lean meats, low-fat cheese, and fresh veggies; these can be used to make soups, salads, sandwiches, and wraps.

• Low-acid sauces like pesto, alfredo, or cheese sauce served over pasta, rice, and noodles that have been prepared with olive oil, herbs, and spices.

• Lean meats, tofu, or beans combined with vegetables like carrots, peas, corn, and zucchini to make stir-fries, curries, and casseroles

• Lean meats like chicken, turkey, or fish that have been roasted, grilled, or baked with herbs, spices, and lemon juice

• Sweetened with honey, maple syrup, or stevia, desserts like cakes, pies, cookies, and muffins prepared with almond flour, whole wheat flour, or oats

Snacks with low-fat yogurt, cheese, or hummus, such as almonds, seeds, dried fruits, granola bars, and crackers

• Drinks prepared with low-acid fruits, like bananas, berries, and mangoes, such as water, coconut water, almond milk, herbal teas, and smoothies.

A low-acid diet can assist you in achieving and sustaining the best possible health and wellness. It is not just a diet, but a way of life.

You may lessen or completely get rid of your acid reflux symptoms by eating a low-acid diet, which will also help with digestion, nutrition, and general health. You and your family can benefit from and find it easy to follow a low-acid diet.

CHAPTER 2

Creating a Low-Acid Pantry

Ingredients You Must Have for Tasty Cooking

One of the difficulties of a low-acid diet is figuring out how to flavor and vary your food without using foods that cause reflux or are rich in acid.

Fortunately, you may create delicious and gratifying foods that neutralize or are low in acid by stocking your cupboard with a variety of items. Several of these components consist of:

• **Spices and herbs:** Without adding acid, they are the simplest and most adaptable ways to give your food flavor and aroma. Herbs and spices including basil, oregano, thyme, rosemary, parsley, cilantro, ginger, turmeric, cumin, coriander, cinnamon, nutmeg, and cardamom can be used either fresh or dried.

Additionally, you can create your own spice and herb mixtures, such za'atar, curry powder, garam masala, and Italian seasoning. Hot and strong herbs and spices (such chile, cayenne, black pepper, garlic, and onion) should not be used as they can irritate your esophagus and cause acid reflux.

• **Olive oil:** A flavorful and healthful fat, olive oil can improve the flavor and texture of your food. Your health and digestion can benefit from the abundance of monounsaturated fatty acids, antioxidants, and anti-inflammatory chemicals found in olive oil.

Because olive oil coats the mucosal lining and shields it from acid damage, it can also help lower the acidity level in your stomach and esophagus. Olive oil can be used in baking, cooking, dressing, and drizzling over meals. Select extra virgin olive oil since it is the best quality and offers the greatest health advantages.

• **Lemon juice:** Due to its acidic composition, lemon juice could seem like an odd addition to a low-acid diet. But because lemon juice can increase the body's synthesis of bicarbonate, a base that can neutralize acid, it can actually have an alkalizing effect on your body.

Additionally, lemon juice can give your food—especially salads, soups, and seafood—a zesty, refreshing flavor. Use lemon juice gently because excessive amounts might still make some people experience acid reflux. For comparable results and flavors, you can also use lime juice, orange juice, or apple cider vinegar in place of lemon juice.

• **Honey:** Honey is a tasty and natural sweetener that you can use to give your food more sweetness and flavor. Because honey has antibacterial, antiviral, and anti-inflammatory qualities that can help treat infections and ease sore throats, it is also good for your health and digestion.

Because honey coats the mucosal lining and shields it from acid damage, it can also help lower the acidity level in your stomach and esophagus. Honey is a useful ingredient for baking, sweetening, and coating food. Because it contains the most nutrients and the fewest additives, go for raw, organic honey.

• **Nuts and seeds**: These wholesome, crunchy items can enhance your meals with protein, fiber, healthy fats, and minerals. Due to their ability to absorb acid and create a protective layer on the mucosal lining, nuts and seeds can also help reduce the amount of acid in your stomach and esophagus. Nuts and seeds can be added to, blended with, or used as a snack.

Select raw, unsalted almonds, walnuts, pistachios, sunflower, pumpkin, and chia seeds among other nuts and seeds. Sesame seeds, cashews, and peanuts are examples of nuts and seeds that should be avoided since they can cause acid reflux.

These are some of the basic ingredients you should always have on hand for flavorful low-acid cooking. You may make delicious, filling, and nutritious recipes that are low in acid or neutralize acid by utilizing these components.

Healthy Kitchen Substitutions

Finding alternatives to or reducing the high-acid or reflux-causing items that are frequently used in baking and cooking is another difficulty while adhering to a low-acid diet.

Thankfully, you may enjoy your favorite foods and recipes without sacrificing your comfort or health by making a lot of wise adjustments in your kitchen.

• **Milk:** A dairy product called milk can make some people experience acid reflux because it relaxes the muscle that keeps acid from flowing back into the esophagus and increases the production of stomach acid. Additionally, milk can result in lactose intolerance, a disorder that causes gas, diarrhea, and bloating because the body is unable to digest the sugar in milk.

Plant-based milks that are lower in acidity and lactose, including rice, oat, or almond milk, can be used in place of milk. Plant-based milks are suitable for baking, cooking, and preparing sauces, soups, and sweets.

• **Cheese:** Similar to milk, cheese is a dairy product that may aggravate acid reflux in certain individuals. Additionally heavy in fat and salt, cheese may exacerbate symptoms of acid reflux.

Low-fat or non-dairy cheeses, like vegan cheese, feta, goat cheese, or mozzarella, can be used in place of cheese because they are lower in fat, acidity, and salt content. Low-fat or nondairy cheeses work well for filling, melting, and topping dishes.

• **Butter:** Because butter relaxes the lower esophageal sphincter and increases stomach acid production, it might cause acid reflux in certain individuals. Additionally, butter may be heavy in cholesterol and saturated fat, both of which are bad for your heart.

Better and more flavorful fats like avocado, coconut, or olive oil can be used in place of butter. For baking, spreading, and cooking, you can use avocado, coconut, or olive oils.

• **Chocolate**: Due to its high fat, caffeine, and theobromine content, which can relax the lower esophageal sphincter and increase stomach acid production, chocolate is a delectable treat that may trigger acid reflux in certain individuals. Additionally, chocolate may include a lot of sugar, which raises the risk of diabetes and weight gain.

Carob, cocoa, or dark chocolate are good alternatives to chocolate because they have less acidity, caffeine, theobromine, fat, and sugar. You can bake, prepare, and consume dishes using carob, cocoa, or dark chocolate.

• **Coffee**: Due to caffeine's ability to both relax the lower esophageal sphincter and accelerate the formation of stomach acid, coffee is a popular beverage that may cause acid reflux in certain individuals.

Additionally, coffee has an acidic quality that might irritate the stomach and esophagus.

Herbal teas with lower acid and caffeine content, including chamomile, ginger, or fennel, can be used in place of coffee. Decaffeinated coffee is another option; it contains half the amount of caffeine as regular coffee. Decaffeinated coffee or herbal teas are good options for unwinding, waking up, and savoring meals.

These are a few of the clever replacements you may make in your kitchen for a lower-acid diet that is more comfortable and healthful. You can lessen or completely get rid of your acid reflux symptoms and enhance your general health and well-being by switching to these alternatives.

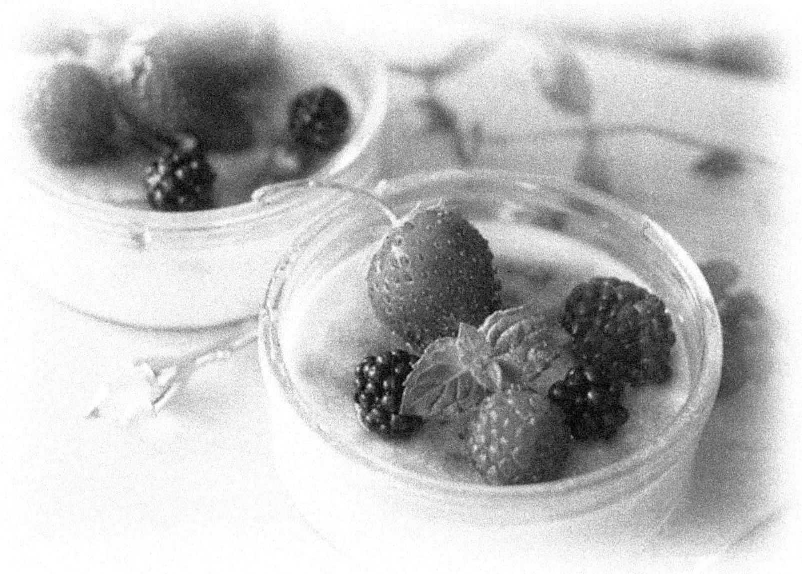

CHAPTER 3

Delectable Morning Meals

Avocado and Spinach with Egg Scrambles

15 minutes of cooking time

Serving size: two

Ingredients

• Four eggs

• One-fourth cup almond milk

• Add pepper and salt to taste.

• One tablespoon of olive oil

• Two cups of young spinach

• Peel and slice one ripe avocado.

Instructions

• Beat the eggs, almond milk, pepper, and salt together thoroughly in a small bowl.

• In a large skillet, heat the olive oil over medium-high heat. Add the spinach and simmer for about 5 minutes, stirring now and again, until the spinach has wilted.

• After lowering the heat to medium-low, cover the spinach with the egg mixture. Cook for about ten minutes, stirring occasionally, or until the eggs are set.

• Spoon the scrambled eggs onto a serving plate, then scatter the avocado slices on top.

Berries and Chia Seed Pudding with Coconut Milk

• Four hours overnight cooking time

• 4 Serving Size

Ingredients

• One-fourth cup chia seeds

• Two cups of coconut milk

• Two tsp honey

• One tsp vanilla extract

• A small amount of salt

• Half a cup of your preferred fresh or frozen fruit

• Combine the chia seeds, coconut milk, honey, vanilla, and salt in a sizable container or bowl. Once the chia seeds have absorbed the liquid and taken on the consistency of pudding, stir thoroughly and place in the refrigerator for at least 4 hours or overnight.

• Spoon pudding into bowls and garnish with berries when ready to serve.

Almond Milk, Spinach, and Banana In A Green Smoothie

5 minutes of cooking time

Serving size: one

Ingredients

• Two cups of young spinach

• One ripe banana, cut into slices and peeled

• A single cup of almond milk

• One tsp almond butter

• One tsp honey

• A couple of ice cubes

• Place the spinach, banana, almond butter, almond milk, honey, and ice in a blender. Adding extra liquid or ice as necessary to modify the consistency, blend until smooth and creamy.

• Transfer the smoothie into a glass, then savor it!

Flaxseeds and Berries with Oatmeal

• 20 minutes of cooking time

Serving size: two

Ingredients

• Full cup rolled oats

• Two water cups

• A small amount of salt

• 1/4 cup of your preferred fresh or frozen fruit

• Two tablespoons flaxseed meal

• Two teaspoons of maple syrup or honey

Instructions

• Bring the water and salt to a boil in a small saucepan. Lower the heat to low and stir in the oats. Simmer for about 15 minutes, stirring now and then, or until the oats are soft and creamy.

• Heat the berries in a small bowl that is safe to use in the microwave for about 30 seconds, or until they are warm and juicy.

• Toast the flaxseeds in a small skillet over medium heat, stirring often, until fragrant and brown, about 5 minutes.

• Spoon the oats into two dishes, then sprinkle the berries, flaxseeds, and maple syrup or honey on top. Have fun!

Herbal Vegetable Omelette

• 20 minutes of cooking time

Serving size: two

Ingredients

• Four eggs

• One-fourth cup almond milk

• Add pepper and salt to taste.

• One tablespoon of olive oil

• 1/4 cup finely chopped onion

• Chopped red bell pepper, 1/4 cup

• 1/4 cup finely chopped mushrooms

• 1/4 cup finely chopped spinach

• Two tablespoons of freshly chopped parsley

• Two tablespoons of freshly chopped basil

• Two tablespoons of optional grated reduced-fat cheese

Instructions

• Beat the eggs, almond milk, pepper, and salt together thoroughly in a small bowl.

• In a large, nonstick skillet, heat the olive oil over medium-high heat. Incorporate the onion, bell pepper, mushroom, and spinach. Cook, stirring often, for approximately ten minutes, or until the veggies become soft.

• After lowering the heat to medium-low, cover the vegetables with the egg mixture. Cook for about 10 minutes, raising the edges with a spatula to allow the raw egg to flow below, or until the omelette is almost set.

• Top half of the omelette with cheese, parsley, and basil, if using. Place the omelette onto a serving platter after folding the second half over the filling. Enjoy after cutting into two pieces!

Pancakes Made Of Quinoa, Berries, and Maple Syrup

• 15 minutes of cooking time

• 4 Serving Size

Ingredients

• One cup prepared quinoa

• A single cup of almond milk

• Two eggs

• Two tsp honey

• One tsp vanilla extract

• One cup flour made from whole wheat

• Two tsp powdered baking

• A small amount of salt

• 1/4 cup of your preferred fresh or frozen fruit

• One-fourth cup of maple syrup

• Place the quinoa, eggs, almond milk, honey, and vanilla in a blender. Process until foamy and smooth.

• Combine the flour, baking powder, and salt in a sizable bowl. Stir the quinoa mixture in thoroughly after adding it.

• Place a skillet or griddle over medium-high heat that has been lightly oiled. Pour approximately 1/4 cup of batter onto the griddle and cook for 3 minutes, or until bubbles start to appear on the surface.

• Allow to cook for an additional two minutes or until golden. Proceed with the leftover batter, yielding approximately 8 pancakes.

• Place the berries and maple syrup in a small microwave-safe bowl and zap for about 30 seconds, or until warm and syrupy.

• Enjoy the pancakes after serving them with the fruit syrup!

Sweet Potato Baked With Corn and Black Beans

• 60 minutes of cooking time

• 4 Serving Size

Ingredients

• Two medium sweet potatoes, cleaned and fork-pierced

• One tablespoon of olive oil

• One-fourth teaspoon cumin

• One-fourth teaspoon paprika

• Add pepper and salt to taste.

• One cup of cooked, drained and rinsed black beans

• Half a cup of frozen or fresh corn kernels

• Two tablespoons of freshly chopped cilantro

• 1/4 cup plain yogurt or low-fat sour cream (optional)

Instructions

• Preheat the oven to 200°C (fan-forced 180°C), and place parchment paper on a baking sheet.

• Halve the sweet potatoes and arrange them cut-side down on the baking sheet that has been preheated. Bake until soft, about 40 to 50 minutes.

• Combine the olive oil, paprika, cumin, salt, and pepper in a small bowl. Combine the corn and black beans with half of the oil mixture in a medium-sized bowl.

• After the sweet potatoes are cooked, turn them over and remove a portion of the meat, leaving a quarter-inch border around the potato. Using a fork, mash the scooped meat and mix in the cilantro. Refill the sweet potato skins with the mixture, then spoon the black bean and corn mixture on top.

• Place the filled sweet potatoes back in the oven and bake for an additional ten minutes, or until well cooked.

• Enjoy the roasted sweet potatoes with yogurt or sour cream, if using!

Chickpea Porridge with Peaches and Chia Seeds

• 30 minutes of cooking time

Serving size: two

Ingredients

• 1/4 cup of drained and washed quinoa

• Two cups almond milk

• Half a cup of chia seeds

• Two teaspoons of maple syrup or honey

• One-fourth teaspoon of cinnamon

• A small amount of salt

• 1/4 cup chopped peaches, either fresh or from a can.

• Two tsp finely chopped almonds

Instructions

• Place the quinoa and one cup of almond milk in a small saucepan and bring to a boil. For around fifteen minutes, or when the quinoa is frothy and soft, lower the heat and simmer it covered.

• Combine the chia seeds, honey, cinnamon, maple syrup, almond milk that's left, and salt in a small bowl. Chia seeds should be refrigerated for a minimum of 15 minutes, or until they have absorbed the liquid and developed a gel-like consistency.

• Heat the peaches in a small bowl that is safe to use in the microwave for 15 seconds or so, or until they are juicy and warm.

• Spoon the quinoa porridge into two dishes, then sprinkle the almonds, peaches, and chia seed pudding over top. Have fun!

Toast Made With Millet with Avocado and Tomato

• 10 minutes of cooking time

Serving size: two

Ingredients

• Four millet bread slices

• One ripe avocado, mashed after peeling

• Add pepper and salt to taste.

• Slicing one medium tomato

• Two tablespoons of freshly chopped basil

• Use a toaster or oven to toast the millet bread until it becomes crisp and brown.

• Add salt and pepper to the mashed avocado in a small bowl.

• Spoon avocado onto bread; add tomato slices and basil on top. Have fun!

Apples Baked with Walnuts and Cinnamon

• 30 minutes of cooking time

• 4 Serving Size

Ingredients

• Cored and sliced four medium apples

• Two teaspoons of maple syrup or honey

• One tsp of cinnamon

• Chopped walnuts, 1/4 cup

Instructions

• Turn the oven on to 180°C (fan-forced at 160°C) and brush a baking dish with a little oil.

• Combine the apple slices, cinnamon, and honey or maple syrup in a big bowl. Place them in the baking dish that has been prepared in a single layer. After the apples, scatter the walnuts on top.

• Bake the apples for 25 to 30 minutes, or until they are bubbly and soft.

• You can serve the baked apples warm or cold, topped with whipped cream or yogurt, if you'd like. Have fun!

CHAPTER 4

Delicious Lunch Recipes

Wraps Of Rainbow Vegetables with Tahini Sauce

15 minutes of cooking time

• 4 Serving Size

Ingredients

• Four tortillas made entirely of whole wheat

• Two cups of purple cabbage, shredded

• Two cups of carrots, shredded

• Two cups of young spinach

• 1/4 cup finely chopped mint, fresh

• One-fourth cup of tahini

• Two teaspoons of juiced lemon

• Two tsp water

• Add pepper and salt to taste.

• Using a small bowl, mix together the tahini, water, lemon juice, salt, and pepper until it becomes creamy and smooth. As necessary, adjust the seasoning and consistency.

• Place the tortillas on a level surface and cover each with around 1 tablespoon of the tahini sauce. Give the edges a one-inch margin.

• Evenly distribute the spinach, carrots, cabbage, and mint among the tortillas. As you carefully roll them up, tuck in the ends.

• Halve the wraps and proceed to serve them with the leftover tahini sauce. Have fun!

Sandwich with Coconut Curry Chickpea Salad

15 minutes of cooking time

• 4 Serving Size

Ingredients

• One-fourth cup plain or vegan yogurt

• Two teaspoons of vegan or traditional mayonnaise

• One tablespoon of curry powder

• Add pepper and salt to taste.

• 1/4 cup of freshly chopped cilantro

• Chopped green onions, 1/4 cup

• One-fourth cup of raisins

• Chopped almonds, 1/4 cup

• One can of washed and drained chickpeas

• Eight whole wheat bread slices

• Four leaves of lettuce

Instructions

• In a sizable bowl, thoroughly mix the yogurt, mayonnaise, curry powder, salt, and pepper. Add the almonds, raisins, green onion, and cilantro and stir.

• Using a fork or a potato masher, finely mash the chickpeas. Toss them to coat after adding them to the yogurt mixture.

• Evenly distribute the chickpea salad among four bread slices. Add the remaining slices of bread and the lettuce leaves on top. Sandwiches should be cut in half to enjoy!

Buddha Bowl Alkaline with Turmeric Tahini Dressing

• Cooking time: fifteen minutes (if pre-roasted veggies and cooked quinoa are used).

• 4 Serving Size

Ingredients

• Two cups prepared quinoa

• Two cups of young spinach

• Two cups of florets of roasted broccoli

• Two cups roasted chunks of sweet potato

• One peeled and sliced avocado

• One-fourth cup of tahini

• Two teaspoons of juiced lemon

• Two tsp water

• One tsp of turmeric

• Add pepper and salt to taste.

• Using a small bowl, mix together the tahini, water, lemon juice, turmeric, salt, and pepper until it becomes creamy and smooth. As necessary, adjust the seasoning and consistency.

• Distribute four bowls of quinoa. Add avocado, sweet potato, broccoli, and spinach on top. Enjoy after adding a drizzle of the turmeric tahini dressing!

Roasted Vegetables with Mediterranean Salmon

30 minutes for cooking time

• 4 Serving Size

Ingredients

• Four 150 g salmon fillets each

• Add pepper and salt to taste.

• Two tsp of olive oil

• Two tsp of dehydrated oregano

• Two tsp of dehydrated thyme

• Four minced garlic cloves

- Four cups of chopped cherry tomatoes

- Two cups of sliced zucchini

- 1/4 cup of freshly chopped parsley

- Two teaspoons of juiced lemon

Instructions

- Preheat the oven to 200°C (fan-forced 180°C), and place parchment paper on a baking sheet.

- Put the salmon fillets on the baking sheet that has been prepared after seasoning them with salt and pepper. One teaspoon each of oregano and thyme should be sprinkled on top of a drizzle of one tablespoon olive oil. Bake for 15 to 20 minutes, or until a fork easily pierces the salmon, indicating that it is done.

- The remaining olive oil and garlic should be heated in a big skillet over medium-high heat. Stir in the zucchini, cherry tomatoes, salt, pepper, and the leftover thyme and oregano. Simmer the veggies for around 15 minutes, stirring now and again, or until they are juicy and soft.

- In a small bowl, thoroughly mix the lemon juice and parsley.

- Drizzle the salmon with the parsley lemon sauce and serve it with the roasted veggies. Have fun!

Curry Soup with Spicy Coconut and Lime Crema

40 minutes of cooking time

• 4 Serving Size

Ingredients

• One tablespoon of coconut oil

• One chopped onion

• Two chopped and peeled carrots

• Two sliced celery stalks

• Two minced garlic cloves

• One tablespoon finely chopped ginger

• Split two tsp curry powder

• One tsp of turmeric

• One-fourth teaspoon of cayenne

• Add pepper and salt to taste.

• Four cups of broth made with vegetables

• One coconut milk can

• Two cups of kale, chopped

• One-fourth cup plain or vegan yogurt

• Two tsp of lemon juice

• Two tablespoons of freshly chopped cilantro

Instructions

• In a large saucepan, heat the coconut oil over medium-high heat. Sauté the onion, carrots, celery, garlic, ginger, turmeric, curry powder, cayenne, salt, and pepper for about ten minutes, or until the onion is tender and the spices are fragrant.

• Include the coconut milk and vegetable broth, then heat the soup until it boils. For about 20 minutes, or until the vegetables are soft, reduce the heat and simmer, covered.

• Add the kale and simmer, stirring, for about 5 minutes, or until wilted.

• In a small bowl, thoroughly mix the yogurt, cilantro, and lime juice.

• Enjoy the soup after serving it with a dollop of the lime crema!

Lettuce Wraps with Tuna Salad

10 minutes of cooking time

• 4 Serving Size

Ingredients

• Two drained and flaked tuna cans

• One-fourth cup plain or vegan yogurt

• Two teaspoons of vegan or traditional mayonnaise

• Two tablespoons of freshly chopped dill

• Add pepper and salt to taste.

• Eight cleaned, dehydrated lettuce leaves

• One-fourth cup finely chopped cucumber

• Chopped red onion, 1/4 cup

Instructions

• Thoroughly mix together the tuna, yogurt, mayonnaise, dill, salt, and pepper in a big bowl.

• Spoon each lettuce leaf with approximately 1/4 cup of the tuna salad. Add some onion and cucumber on top, then savor!

<u>Tabouli made of Quinoa and Roasted Vegetables</u>

30 minutes for cooking time

• 4 Serving Size

Ingredients

• Two cups prepared quinoa

• Two cups of chopped cherry tomatoes

• Two cups of florets of cauliflower

• Two tsp of olive oil

• Add pepper and salt to taste.

• 1/4 cup of freshly chopped parsley

• 1/4 cup finely chopped mint, fresh

• Two teaspoons of juiced lemon

Instructions

• Preheat the oven to 200°C (fan-forced 180°C), and place parchment paper on a baking sheet.

• Combine the cauliflower and cherry tomatoes with the olive oil, salt, and pepper in a big bowl. Arrange them on the prepared baking sheet in a single layer. Roast the vegetables for 25 to 30 minutes, or until they are soft and browned.

• In a small bowl, thoroughly mix the lemon juice, mint, and parsley.

• Combine the quinoa, roasted veggies, and herb dressing in a sizable serving bowl. Have fun!

Lentil Soup with Lemon and Dill

30 minutes for cooking time

• 4 Serving Size

Ingredients

• One tablespoon of olive oil

• One chopped onion

• Two chopped and peeled carrots

• Two sliced celery stalks

• Two minced garlic cloves

• One teaspoon of cumin

• One-fourth teaspoon of turmeric

• Add pepper and salt to taste.

• Four cups of broth made with vegetables

• Two water cups

• One cup of washed and drained red lentils

• A pair of bay leaves

• One-fourth cup of lemon juice

• Two tablespoons of freshly chopped dill

Instructions

• In a large saucepan, heat the coconut oil over medium-high heat. Sauté the onion, carrots, celery, garlic, cumin, turmeric, salt, and pepper for about ten minutes, or until the onion is tender and the spices are fragrant.

• Bring the soup to a boil after adding the lentils, water, vegetable broth, and bay leaves. For about 20 minutes, or until the lentils are tender and mushy, reduce the heat and simmer, covered.

• Toss in the dill and lemon juice after discarding the bay leaves. As necessary, adjust the seasoning.   .

• If preferred, serve the soup hot or cold with bread or crackers. Have fun!

Quinoa and Roasted Asparagus with Salmon

30 minutes for cooking time

• 4 Serving Size

Ingredients

• Four 150 g salmon fillets each

• Add pepper and salt to taste.

• Two tsp honey

• Two tablespoons of sesame oil

• One tsp of sesame oil

• One tablespoon finely chopped ginger

• One minced garlic clove

• Two cups of asparagus, quartered and cleaned

• Two cups prepared quinoa

• Two tablespoons of freshly chopped parsley

Instructions

• Preheat the oven to 200°C (fan-forced 180°C), and place parchment paper on a baking sheet.

• Put the salmon fillets on the baking sheet that has been prepared after seasoning them with salt and pepper. Mix the honey, soy sauce, sesame oil, ginger, and garlic thoroughly in a small bowl.

• Transfer half of the sauce to the salmon fillets; set aside remaining sauce for another time.

• Salmon should be baked for 15 to 20 minutes, or until it is cooked through and flake readily when tested with a fork.

• Saute the asparagus in a big skillet over medium-high heat for approximately ten minutes, or until it's crisp-tender. Season with salt and pepper.

• Heat the remaining sauce in a small saucepan over low heat for about five minutes, stirring regularly, until it thickens slightly.

• Present the quinoa and roasted asparagus with the fish. Add a drizzle of sauce and garnish with parsley.

Alkaline Green Smoothie

5 minutes of cooking time

Serving size: one

Ingredients

• Two cups of young spinach

• One chopped and peeled cucumber

• One chopped and cored green apple

• Half an avocado, cut and peeled

• One-fourth cup of mint leaves, raw

• Two teaspoons of juiced lemon

• One tablespoon of maple syrup or honey

• A couple of ice cubes

Instructions

• The spinach, cucumber, apple, avocado, mint, lemon juice, honey or maple syrup, and ice should all be combined in a blender. Adding extra liquid or ice as necessary to modify the consistency, blend until smooth and creamy.

• Transfer the smoothie into a glass, then savor it!

CHAPTER 5

Satisfying Dinners

Roasted Chicken with Lemon Herbs and Root Vegetables

• 90 minutes of cooking

• 4 servings per size

Ingredients

• One 1.5 kilogram entire chicken

• Add pepper and salt to taste.

• 4 peeled and crushed garlic cloves

• One lemon, cut in half

• Four fresh rosemary sprigs

• Four fresh thyme sprigs

• Two tsp of olive oil

• Four cups of finely diced root vegetables, including turnips, potatoes, carrots, and parsnips

• Turn the oven on to 200°C (fan-forced 180°C), and brush a baking dish with a little oil.

• Use paper towels to pat the chicken dry after rinsing it. Put some salt and pepper in the chicken cavity and then load it with two cloves of garlic, one half of a lemon, two sprigs of rosemary, and two sprigs of thyme. Use kitchen twine to secure the legs together, then tuck the wings under the body.

• After rubbing olive oil all over its skin, place the chicken in the baking dish that has been prepared. Drizzle the chicken with the juice from the remaining lemon half and season with additional salt and pepper.

• Arrange the chicken with the remaining garlic cloves, thyme sprigs, and rosemary sprigs all around it.

• For one hour, bake the chicken, basting it periodically with pan juices.

• Combine the root veggies with a little bit of the pan juices, salt, and pepper in a big bowl. Put the baking dish back in the oven after arranging them around the chicken. Bake for a further half hour, or until the veggies are soft and the chicken is golden and cooked through.

• After transferring the chicken to a chopping board, give it ten minutes to rest. After carving the chicken, serve it with more pan juices and the roasted vegetables.

Alkaline Salmon Paired With Asparagus and Quinoa Salad

• 30 minutes for cooking

• 4 servings per size

Ingredients

• Four 150 g salmon fillets each

• Add pepper and salt to taste.

• Two tsp honey

• Two tablespoons of sesame oil

• One tsp of sesame oil

• One tablespoon finely chopped ginger

• One minced garlic clove

• Two cups prepared quinoa

• Two tablespoons of freshly chopped parsley

• Two cups of asparagus, quartered and cleaned

• Preheat the oven to 200°C (fan-forced 180°C), and place parchment paper on a baking sheet.

• Put the salmon fillets on the baking sheet that has been prepared after seasoning them with salt and pepper. Mix the honey, soy sauce, sesame oil, ginger, and garlic thoroughly in a small bowl. Transfer half of the sauce to the salmon fillets; set aside remaining sauce for another time.

• Salmon should be baked for 15 to 20 minutes, or until it is cooked through and flake readily when tested with a fork.

• Saute the asparagus in a big skillet over medium-high heat for approximately ten minutes, or until it's crisp-tender. Season with salt and pepper.

• Heat the remaining sauce in a small saucepan over low heat for about five minutes, stirring regularly, until it thickens slightly.

• Place the quinoa, parsley, and a portion of the sauce in a big serving bowl.

• Present the asparagus and quinoa pilaf alongside the salmon. Enjoy and drizzle with more sauce!

Shrimp with Coconut Curry and Zucchini Noodles

- 40 minutes for cooking

- 4 servings per size

Ingredients

- One tablespoon of coconut oil

- One chopped onion

- Two minced garlic cloves

- One tablespoon finely chopped ginger

- Split two tsp curry powder

- One-fourth teaspoon of cayenne

- Add pepper and salt to taste.

- One coconut milk can

- One-fourth cup of vegetable broth

- 1/4 cup of freshly chopped cilantro

- 1/4 cup of freshly chopped basil

- One-fourth cup lime juice

- 500 grams of deveined and peeled shrimp

• Four medium zucchini, thinly sliced or spiralled

• In a large saucepan, heat the coconut oil over medium-high heat. Sauté the onion, garlic, ginger, curry powder, cayenne, salt, and pepper for about 10 minutes, or until the onion is tender and the spices are fragrant.

• Add the lime juice, cilantro, basil, coconut milk, and vegetable broth. Then, bring the sauce to a boil. Lower the temperature and let it simmer, covered, for around 15 minutes, stirring now and again, until it thickens somewhat.

• Add the shrimp and simmer, stirring, for about 10 minutes, or until they become pink and opaque.

• Cook the zucchini noodles in a large pot of boiling water for about 5 minutes, or until they are soft. After draining, rinse with cold water.

• Arrange the noodles made of zucchini and top with the shrimp and sauce. Savor!

Sweet Potato Mash with Turkey Meatloaf

- 60 minutes of cooking

- 4 servings per size

Ingredients

- 500 grams of turkey ground lean.

- One-fourth cup of oatmeal

- One-fourth cup almond milk

- Just one egg

- Two tablespoons of freshly chopped parsley

- Two tablespoons of freshly chopped sage

- Add pepper and salt to taste.

- Two tsp honey

- Two tablespoons of sesame oil

- One tablespoon vinegar made from apple cider

- Four medium-sized sweet potatoes, diced and peeling

- Two tsp of olive oil

- Two tsp pure maple syrup

Instructions

• Turn the oven on to 180°C (fan-forced to 160°C) and brush a loaf pan gently with oil.

• Combine the turkey, oats, egg, almond milk, sage, parsley, and salt and pepper in a big bowl. Blend thoroughly and form into a loaf. Smooth the top and place in the prepared pan.

• In a small bowl, thoroughly mix the vinegar, soy sauce, and honey. Transfer half of the glaze onto the meatloaf; set aside remaining glaze for another time.

• Bake the meatloaf for forty to fifty minutes, or until it is brown and cooked through. Halfway through the baking time, baste with the leftover glaze.

• Boil the sweet potatoes in a big saucepan for about 20 minutes, or until they are tender. Empty and put back into the pot. Once the sweet potatoes are smooth and creamy, mash them with the olive oil, maple syrup, salt, and pepper.

• Enjoy the meatloaf served with the sweet potato mash!

Creamy Almond Milk Mushroom Soup

• 40 minutes for cooking

• 4 servings per size

Ingredients

• Two tsp of olive oil

• One chopped onion

• Two minced garlic cloves

• Four cups of sliced button, cremini, or shiitake mushrooms

• Add pepper and salt to taste.

• Four cups of broth made with vegetables

• Two cups almond milk

• Two teaspoons corn flour

• Two tsp water

• Two tablespoons of freshly chopped parsley

Instructions

• Heat the olive oil in a large pot over medium-high heat. Sauté the onion, garlic, mushrooms, salt, and pepper for about 15 minutes, or until the onion is tender and the mushrooms are browned.

• Pour in the almond milk and vegetable broth, then heat the soup until it boils. Lower the temperature and let the mushrooms cook, covered, for around 15 minutes, stirring now and then, until they become soft.

• Combine the cornstarch and water in a small bowl and whisk until smooth. After adding the cornstarch mixture to the soup, stir it and continue cooking for about five minutes, or until the soup thickens somewhat.

• Garnish the soup with parsley and serve it hot or cold.

Baked Tilapia with Tomatoes and Herbs

• 30 minutes for cooking

• 4 servings per size

Ingredients

• Four 150 g fillets of tilapia

• Add pepper and salt to taste.

• Two tsp of olive oil

• Two tsp of dehydrated oregano

• Two tsp preserved basil

• Four minced garlic cloves

• Two cups of chopped cherry tomatoes

• Two tablespoons of freshly chopped parsley

Instructions

• Preheat the oven to 200°C (fan-forced 180°C), and place parchment paper on a baking sheet.

• Put the tilapia fillets on the baking sheet that has been prepared after seasoning them with salt and pepper. Add a drizzle of 1 tablespoon olive oil and a dusting of 1 teaspoon each of oregano and basil. Fish should flake easily with a fork and be cooked through after 15 to 20 minutes in the oven.

• The remaining olive oil and garlic should be heated in a big skillet over medium-high heat. Incorporate the cherry tomatoes, salt, pepper, and the leftover basil and oregano. Simmer for approximately 15 minutes, stirring now and again, or until the tomatoes are luscious and tender.

• Garnish the fish with parsley and serve it with the tomato sauce. Have fun!

Pasta Verde with Lentils and Lemon Zest

• 25 minutes for cooking

• 4 servings per size

Ingredients

• Four cups cooked spaghetti with lentils

• Two tsp of olive oil

• One chopped onion

• Two minced garlic cloves

• Two cups of florets of broccoli

• Two cups thinly sliced mushroom

• Two cups of young spinach

• Add pepper and salt to taste.

• One-fourth cup of vegetable broth

• Two teaspoons of juiced lemon

• One tsp lemon zest

• Two tablespoons of freshly chopped basil

Instructions

• Cook the lentil pasta in a large saucepan of boiling water until al dente, following the directions on the package. Empty and put back into the pot.

• Heat the olive oil in a large skillet over medium-high heat. Sauté the onion, garlic, broccoli, and mushrooms for about 15 minutes, or until the onion is soft and the vegetables are crisp-tender.

• Cook, stirring, for about 5 minutes, or until the spinach is wilted and the sauce is slightly thickened. Add the spinach, salt, pepper, vegetable broth, lemon juice, and lemon zest.

• Include the basil and mix well.

• Enjoy the pasta served with the vegetable sauce!

Brown Rice and Vegetables in a Stir-Fried Chicken Dish

• 30 minutes for cooking

• 4 servings per size

Ingredients

• 500 grams of thinly sliced chicken breast

• Add pepper and salt to taste.

- Two teaspoons corn flour

- Two tablespoons of sesame oil

- Two tsp honey

- One tsp of sesame oil

- One tablespoon finely chopped ginger

- One minced garlic clove

- Vegetable oil, two tablespoons

- Two cups of carrots, sliced

- A pair of cups snow peas

- Two cups of brown rice, cooked.

- Two tablespoons of freshly chopped cilantro

Instructions

- Toss the chicken with the cornstarch in a big bowl after seasoning it with salt and pepper. Mix the soy sauce, honey, sesame oil, ginger, and garlic thoroughly in a small bowl.

- Heat the vegetable oil in a big skillet or wok over high heat. Stir-fry the chicken for about 15 minutes, or until it is brown and cooked through. After moving the chicken to a platter, reheat it.

• Stir-fry the carrots and snow peas in the same skillet or wok for about ten minutes, or until they are crisp-tender. Bring the sauce to a boil after adding it. Simmer the sauce for approximately five minutes, stirring occasionally, on low heat until it thickens slightly.

• Arrange the veggies and chicken on top of the rice, then garnish with cilantro.

Scampi with Shrimp and Zucchini Noodles

• 25 minutes for cooking

• 4 servings per size

Ingredients

• 500 grams of deveined and peeled shrimp

• Add pepper and salt to taste.

• Two tsp of olive oil

• Four minced garlic cloves

• Fourteen milligrams of red pepper flakes

• 1/4 cup of veggie broth or white wine

• Two teaspoons of juiced lemon

• Two tablespoons of freshly chopped parsley

• Four medium zucchini, thinly sliced or spiralized

Instructions

• After adding salt and pepper to the shrimp, set them aside.

• Heat the olive oil in a large skillet over medium-high heat. Sauté the garlic and red pepper flakes for about two minutes, or until fragrant.

• Add the shrimp and simmer, stirring, for about 10 minutes, or until they become pink and opaque.

• Include the parsley, lemon juice, and wine or broth and bring to a boil. After lowering the heat, simmer the sauce for approximately five minutes while stirring occasionally.

• Cook the zucchini noodles in a large pot of boiling water for about 5 minutes, or until they are soft. After draining, rinse with cold water.

• Arrange the noodles made of zucchini and top with the shrimp and sauce. Savor!

CHAPTER 6

Snacks and Sweet Desserts

Cookies Made With Almond Flour and Dark Chocolate Chips

• 20 minutes for cooking

• 16 cookies, serving size

Ingredients

• Almond flour, two cups

• One-fourth teaspoon of baking soda

• A small amount of salt

• 1/4 cup melted coconut oil

• One-fourth cup of maple syrup or honey

• One tsp vanilla extract

½ cup of chips made of dark chocolate

Instructions

• Adjust the oven temperature to 180°C (fan-forced to 160°C) and place parchment paper on a baking sheet.

• In a sizable bowl, thoroughly mix the baking soda, salt, and almond flour.

• Combine the vanilla, honey (or maple syrup), and coconut oil in a small bowl and whisk until smooth and creamy.

• Combine the wet and dry ingredients, stirring to combine them into a dough. Add the chocolate chips and fold.

• Drop, allowing space between each one, by rounded tablespoonful onto the baking sheet that has been prepared. Using a spatula or your fingers, gently flatten.

• Bake for ten to twelve minutes, or until the edges are firm and brown. After 10 minutes of cooling on the baking sheet, move the cookies to a wire rack to finish cooling.

Granola and Fruit Paired With a Coconut Yogurt Parfait

• 10 minutes for cooking

• 4 Serving Size

Ingredients

• Two cups of vegan or coconut yogurt

• Two cups of cereal

• Two cups of your preferred fresh or frozen fruit, such as mangoes, bananas, or berries

Instructions

• Arrange the fruit, granola, and yogurt in four glasses or jars, switching between them as you please. If you'd like, you can also pour some maple syrup or honey over the layers.

• Enjoy the parfaits immediately away, or refrigerate until ready to serve.

Walnut and Dried Cranberry Oatmeal Cookies

• 20 minutes for cooking

• 24 cookies, serving size

Ingredients

• 1/4 cup softened coconut oil

• One-fourth cup of maple syrup or honey

• Just one egg

• One tsp vanilla extract

• One and a half cups rolled oats

• One-half cup whole wheat flour

• One-half tsp baking soda

• A small amount of salt

• Dried cranberries, 1/4 cup

• Chopped walnuts, 1/4 cup

Instructions

• Adjust the oven temperature to 180°C (fan-forced to 160°C) and place parchment paper on a baking sheet.

• Using a large bowl, beat together the coconut oil and maple syrup or honey until frothy and light. Beat well after adding the egg and vanilla.

• In a small basin, thoroughly mix the flour, baking soda, oats, and salt. Stirring until a dough forms, add the dry ingredients to the wet ones. Stir in the walnuts and cranberries.

• Leaving some space between each drop, place by rounded teaspoonful onto the baking sheet that has been prepared. Using a spatula or your fingers, gently flatten.

• Bake for 8 to 10 minutes, until the edges become firm and brown. After 10 minutes of cooling on the baking sheet, move the cookies to a wire rack to finish cooling.

Pumpkin Muffins with Spice and Pecan Crumble

• 35 minutes for cooking

12 Muffins, Serving Size

Ingredients

- Almond flour, two cups

- One-fourth cup coconut sugar

- Two tsp powdered baking

- One tsp of cinnamon

- One-half tsp nutmeg

- One-fourth teaspoon of ginger

- One-fourth teaspoon of cloves

- A small amount of salt

- One-third cup pureed pumpkin

- 1/4 cup melted coconut oil

- Two eggs

- One tsp vanilla extract

- Chopped pecans, 1/4 cup

- Oats, two tablespoons

- Two tsp pure maple syrup

Instructions

- Pre-heat the oven to 180°C (or 160°C if using a fan) and insert paper liners into a muffin pan.

- In a sizable bowl, thoroughly mix the almond flour, coconut sugar, baking powder, cloves, ginger, nutmeg, cinnamon, and salt.

- In a small bowl, mix together the eggs, vanilla, coconut oil, and pumpkin puree until well combined and creamy.

- Combine the wet and dry ingredients, stirring to combine them into a batter.

- Combine the oats, maple syrup, and pecans in a small bowl and stir until evenly distributed.

- Evenly distribute the batter into the muffin cups, filling them to about 3/4 of the way. Gently push the crumbled pecans into the batter to ensure they stick.

- When a toothpick is placed in the center, the baked food should come out clean after 20 to 25 minutes. After 10 minutes of cooling in the muffin pan, move the muffins to a wire rack to finish cooling.

Rice Cakes with Sprouts and Avocado

- 10 minutes for cooking

- 4 Serving Size

Ingredients

- Four cakes of rice

- One ripe avocado, mashed after peeling

- Add pepper and salt to taste.

- 1/4 cup of sprouting alfalfa

- Two tablespoons of freshly chopped chives

Instructions

- Add salt and pepper to the mashed avocado in a small bowl.

- Top the rice cakes with the avocado spread and the chives and sprouts.

Banana Bread with Dark Chocolate Chips and Almond Flour

• 60 minutes of cooking

Ten slices are the serving size.

Ingredients

• Three ripe bananas, mashed after peeling

• One-fourth cup of maple syrup or honey

• Two eggs

• One tsp vanilla extract

• Almond flour, two cups

• One baking soda tsp

• A small amount of salt

½ cup of chips made of dark chocolate

Instructions

• Turn the oven on to 180°C (fan-forced to 160°C) and brush a loaf pan gently with oil.

• In a sizable bowl, thoroughly mix the eggs, vanilla, honey or maple syrup, and bananas.

• In a separate basin, thoroughly mix the baking soda, salt, and almond flour. When a batter develops, add the dry ingredients to the wet components and whisk. Add the chocolate chips and fold.

• Transfer the mixture into the ready pan and level the surface. When a toothpick inserted in the center comes out clean, bake for 40 to 50 minutes. After allowing the bread to cool in the pan for ten minutes, move it to a wire rack to finish cooling.

Handmade Trail Mix with Dried Fruit, Nuts, and Seeds

• 25 minutes for cooking

16-ounce serving size

Ingredients

• One cup uncooked almonds

• One cup uncooked walnuts

• One-half cup uncooked pumpkin seeds

• One-half cup uncooked sunflower seeds

• One-fourth cup of maple syrup or honey

• One-fourth teaspoon of salt

- One-fourth teaspoon of cinnamon

- One-fourth teaspoon nutmeg

- One cup of cranberries, dried

- One cup of chopped dried apricots

Instructions

- Adjust the oven temperature to 180°C (fan-forced to 160°C) and place parchment paper on a baking sheet.

- In a sizable bowl, thoroughly mix the almonds, walnuts, pumpkin seeds, and sunflower seeds with the salt, nutmeg, cinnamon, and honey or maple syrup.

- On the baking sheet that has been prepared, distribute the nut and seed mixture in a single layer. Bake, stirring regularly, for 15 to 20 minutes, or until golden and crisp.

- After allowing the trail mix to cool fully on the baking sheet, move it to a sizable bowl. Add the apricots and cranberries and stir.

- For up to two weeks, keep the trail mix refrigerated or at room temperature in an airtight container.

Honey-Baked Pears with Walnuts

• 30 minutes for cooking

• 4 Serving Size

Ingredients

• Four ripe pears, cored and halved.

• Two teaspoons of maple syrup or honey

• One-fourth teaspoon of cinnamon

• Chopped walnuts, 1/4 cup

• 1/4 cup of vegan or plain yogurt, if desired

Instructions

• Turn the oven on to 180°C (fan-forced at 160°C) and brush a baking dish with a little oil

• Place the pear halves cut-side up in the baking dish that has been preheated. Sprinkle with the walnuts and cinnamon, then drizzle with honey or maple syrup.

• Bake the pears for twenty to thirty minutes, or until they are soft and caramelized.

• You can serve the pears cold or warm, with yogurt if you'd like.

Spices & Herbs in Roasted Chickpeas

• 30 minutes for cooking

8-piece serving size

Ingredients

• Two cans of rinsed and drained chickpeas

• Two tsp of olive oil

• Add pepper and salt to taste.

• Two tsp of dehydrated oregano

• Two tsp of rosemary, dried

• One-fourth teaspoon of cayenne

Instructions

• Preheat the oven to 200°C (fan-forced 180°C), and place parchment paper on a baking sheet.

• Using paper towels, pat dry the chickpeas and then transfer them to a large bowl. Mix thoroughly to coat with the olive oil, salt, pepper, oregano, rosemary, and cayenne.

• Arrange the chickpeas on the baking sheet that has been preheated in a single layer. Bake, stirring the pan regularly, until the chickpeas are crisp and brown, 25 to 30 minutes.

• After allowing the chickpeas on the baking sheet to cool slightly, move them to a bowl or an airtight container. Savor it as a salad dressing or as a snack.

Bark of Dark Chocolate with Cranberries and Almonds

• 10 minutes of cooking time (plus 2 hours of refrigeration)

16-ounce serving size

Ingredients

• 300 grams of chopped dark chocolate

• Almond slices, 1/4 cup

• Dried cranberries, 1/4 cup

Instructions

• Use parchment paper to line a baking sheet.

• Melt and smooth out the chocolate in a bowl that is safe to use in the microwave by heating it for 30 seconds at a time, stirring in between.

• Transfer the chocolate onto the baking sheet that has been ready and use a spatula to spread it into a thin layer. Almonds and cranberries should be sprinkled over top; gently press to adhere.

• Chill the chocolate bark for about two hours, or until it solidifies. Split apart and savor!

Quinoa, Berries, and Coconut Milk in a Parfait

• 10 minutes for cooking

• 4 Serving Size

Ingredients

• Two cups prepared quinoa

• Two cups of vegan or plain yogurt

• Two cups of your preferred fresh or frozen fruit

• One-fourth cup of coconut milk

• Two teaspoons of maple syrup or honey

• Arrange the quinoa, yogurt, and berries in four glasses or jars, mixing and matching as desired. If you'd like, you can also pour some maple syrup or honey over the layers.

• In a small bowl, thoroughly whisk together the coconut milk and maple syrup or honey.

• Enjoy the parfaits after drizzling them with the coconut milk mixture!

Energy Bites with Dates, Nuts, and Seeds

• 20 minutes of cooking time (plus two hours of refrigeration)

• 24 serving size

Ingredients

• One cup of dates with pits

• Half a cup uncooked almonds

• Half a cup uncooked cashews

• One-fourth cup of sunflower seeds

• One-fourth cup of pumpkin seeds

• Half a cup of chia seeds

• Two tablespoons flaxseed meal

• One-fourth teaspoon of salt

• Two tsp water

Instructions

• Pulse the dates in a food processor until a sticky paste forms. Move to a sizable bowl and reserve.

• Process the almonds, cashews, pumpkin, sunflower, chia, and flaxseeds, as well as the salt, until finely chopped using the food processor. Incorporate them thoroughly with the date paste.

• Work the dough until it comes together after adding the water. As necessary, add more water if it's too dry. Add extra nuts or seeds as necessary if it's too moist.

• Using a baking sheet covered with parchment paper, shape the mixture into bite-sized balls. Put in the fridge for two hours or until firm.

14 Days Meal Plan for Low Acid Diet

Day 1

- **Breakfast**: Scrambled Eggs with Spinach and Avocado
- **Lunch**: Rainbow Veggie Wraps with Tahini Sauce
- **Dinner**: Lemon Herb Roasted Chicken with Root Vegetables
- **Snack**: Baked Apples with Cinnamon and Walnuts

Day 2

- **Breakfast**: Coconut Milk Chia Seed Pudding with Berries
- **Lunch**: Coconut Curry Chickpea Salad Sandwich
- **Dinner**: Alkaline Salmon with Quinoa Pilaf and Asparagus
- **Snack**: Dates Stuffed with Almond Butter and Coconut

Day 3

- **Breakfast**: Green Smoothie with Spinach, Banana, and Almond Milk
- **Lunch**: Alkaline Buddha Bowl with Turmeric Tahini Dressing
- **Dinner**: Coconut Curry Shrimp with Zucchini Noodles
- **Snack**: Banana "Nice" Cream with Berries

- **Breakfast**: Oatmeal with Berries and Flaxseeds
- **Lunch**: Mediterranean Salmon with Roasted Vegetables
- **Dinner**: Turkey Meatloaf with Sweet Potato Mash
- **Snack**: Mango Lassi with Coconut Milk and Cardamom

Day 5

- **Breakfast**: Vegetable Omelette with Herbs
- **Lunch**: Spicy Coconut Curry Soup with Lime Crema
- **Dinner**: Creamy Mushroom Soup with Almond Milk
- **Snack**: Almond Flour Cookies with Dark Chocolate Chips

Day 6

- **Breakfast**: Quinoa Pancakes with Berries and Maple Syrup
- **Lunch**: Tuna Salad Lettuce Wraps
- **Dinner**: Baked Tilapia with Herbs and Tomatoes
- **Snack**: Coconut Yogurt Parfait with Granola and Fruit

Day 7

- **Breakfast**: Baked Sweet Potato with Black Beans and Corn
- **Lunch**: Quinoa Tabouli with Roasted Vegetables
- **Dinner**: Lentil Pasta Primavera with Lemon Zest
- **Snack**: Oatmeal Cookies with Dried Cranberries and Walnuts

- **Breakfast**: Quinoa Porridge with Chia Seeds and Peaches
- **Lunch**: Lentil Soup with Lemon and Dill
- **Dinner**: Chicken Stir-Fry with Vegetables and Brown Rice
- **Snack**: Baked Sweet Potato Fries with Cinnamon and Maple Syrup

Day 9

- **Breakfast**: Millet Toast with Avocado and Tomato
- **Lunch**: Salmon with Roasted Asparagus and Quinoa
- **Dinner**: Shrimp Scampi with Zucchini Noodles
- **Snack**: Spiced Pumpkin Muffins with Pecan Crumble

Day 10

- **Breakfast**: Baked Apples with Cinnamon and Walnuts
- **Lunch**: Alkaline Green Smoothie
- **Dinner**: Roasted Cauliflower Steaks with Tahini Sauce
- **Snack**: Rice Cakes with Avocado and Sprouts

Day 11

- **Breakfast**: Scrambled Eggs with Spinach and Avocado
- **Lunch**: Rainbow Veggie Wraps with Tahini Sauce
- **Dinner**: Lemon Herb Roasted Chicken with Root Vegetables
- **Snack**: Banana Bread with Almond Flour and Dark Chocolate

Day 12

- **Breakfast**: Coconut Milk Chia Seed Pudding with Berries
- **Lunch**: Coconut Curry Chickpea Salad Sandwich
- **Dinner**: Alkaline Salmon with Quinoa Pilaf and Asparagus
- **Snack**: Homemade Trail Mix with Nuts, Seeds, and Dried Fruit

Day 13

- **Breakfast**: Green Smoothie with Spinach, Banana, and Almond Milk
- **Lunch**: Alkaline Buddha Bowl with Turmeric Tahini Dressing
- **Dinner**: Coconut Curry Shrimp with Zucchini Noodles
- **Snack**: Chia Seed Pudding with Coconut Milk and Mango

Day 14

- **Breakfast**: Oatmeal with Berries and Flaxseeds
- **Lunch**: Mediterranean Salmon with Roasted Vegetables
- **Dinner**: Turkey Meatloaf with Sweet Potato Mash
- **Snack**: Baked Pears with Honey and Walnuts

CONCLUSION

We sincerely thank you for embarking on this delicious journey toward a healthier, more vibrant self as you approach the last pages of the Low Acid Diet Cookbook. It has been our pleasure to lead you on a gastronomic journey that puts health first without sacrificing the enjoyment of food.

Our goal is for this cookbook to serve as more than just a guide of recipes; we want it to inspire positive transformation in your life. Your journey is our success, whether you've found a new favorite breakfast, perfected a dinner party menu, or just experienced the joy of intentionally fuelling your body.

We hope you will continue to delve into the world of low-acid cooking as we say goodbye. Let this experience serve as a springboard for a lifestyle that balances flavor with well-being. You can now use your kitchen as a blank canvas to prepare meals that nourish your body and soul.

Your positive Opinion Counts

We encourage you to tell others about your cooking adventures if this cookbook has brought a little joy into your everyday. Your encouraging comments not only make us smile, but they also encourage other readers to experience the advantages and delights of living a low-acid lifestyle.

By writing a favorable feedback on the book's purchase site, you may assist us in forming future editions and encourage others to pursue wellbeing. Your opinions are very valuable, and we look forward to hearing from you.

I hope you have

many more delicious

meals in the future,

as well as good health

and happiness!